The Bride's Guide
Less Stress

A Quick & Easy Way to
Reduce Your Wedding Stress

by

Carol L Rickard, LCSW

America's Ultimate Stress Expert

As Featured:

The Bride's Guide to Less Stress
by Carol L Rickard, LCSW

© 2019 Carol L Rickard   All Rights Reserved

All rights reserved. No part of this book may be reproduced for resale, redistribution, or any other purposes (including but not limited to eBooks, pamphlets, articles, video or audiotapes, & handouts or slides for lectures or workshops). Permission to reproduce these materials for those and any other purposes must be obtained in writing from the author.

The author & publisher of this book do not dispense medical advice nor prescribe the use of this material as a form of treatment. The author & publisher are not engaged in rendering psychological, medical, or other professional services. The purpose of this material is educational only.

ISBN: 978-1-947745-20-9 (paperback)
ISBN: 978-1-947745-16-2 (Kindle)
Library of Congress Control Number: 2019911100

Published by:

Well YOUniversity Publications
A Division of Well YOUniversity, LLC
5 Zion Rd.
Hopewell, NJ 08525
888 LIFE TOOLS (543-3866)
www.WellYOUniversity.com

What will you get out of this book?

- A better understanding of WHY you must take action to reduce & manage your wedding stress.

- A simple & practical system that will decrease your STRESS levels in just 60 seconds or less!

- A beautiful wedding you can now enjoy because you know how to *keep STRESS from ruining it!*

Table of Contents

Why I Wrote This Book	1
Welcome	3
Getting Started	6
About the Book	10

Part 1: It's In The Cards!!

It's In the Cards	16
Tracking Progress	21

Part 2: Now You See It!

#1 – Root Beer	30
#2 – The Tub	39

Part 3: Now You Don't!

WHAT To Do	46
HOW To Do It - Step 1	53
HOW To Do It - Step 2	67
Wrap Up	81
Bonus - The Serenity Stress Tool	89
DO*60* System *Mini Poster*	93
Keys to Success *Mini Poster*	95
The Stressometer™ *Mini Poster*	97
Carol's Other Resources	101

Sign Up For...

This 5 minute video newsletter will give you more tips, tools, & rules for taking control of...

STRESS!

Sign up at:

StressYOUniversity.com/Stress-Talk

Why I Wrote This Book

There are certain **milestones** we get to experience ONLY once…

 1st day of school

H.S. Graduation

Getting married

1st child

STRESS -

has the **POWER** to *ruin them all.*

This is what happened to me at my high school graduation.

The stress led to a horrible **migraine** &

I couldn't enjoy any part of it…

 NOT the ceremony

NOT the moment

NOT the party

IT SUCKED….

I've spent **25+** years

teaching people in hospitals

how to **take control** of stress.

My dream:

Teach these *same skills* to everyone.

Brides are the first ones I thought of!

Welcome

Stress comes wrapped up in

some pretty amazing packages!

Weddings happen to be one of them!

It's one of the **most joyful & special** days

and yet,

one of the **MOST** *stressful* as well!

If you are reading this , there is

one thing I know for sure about you…

You are either...

a bride to be

OR

family / friend of a bride to be!

Whichever it is –

I am glad you are here!

There is NO *shortage* when it comes to **wedding stress!**

 The bride, the groom,

the wedding party, the families...

There's plenty to go around & be shared!

The problem is…

when **Stress** is not managed,

it has the *power to ruin* a lot of things…

health

    relationships

        hopes

            dreams

                &… weddings.

It is my sincere hope you will take &

use what you learn in this book!

You will either manage your stress

or

IT WILL MANAGE YOU!

Getting Started

Let me ask you a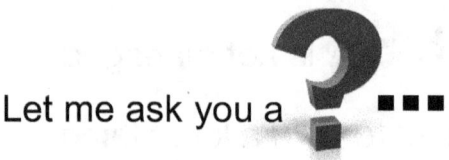

What if you could learn how to

eliminate stress in just **60** *seconds*?

Would you want to know?

If the answer is **"yes"**

than just keep on reading!

You are about to learn a **revolutionary approach** to managing your stress.

This approach will put YOU in *control of stress* once & for all.

It may seem like it is too good to be true –

But *it isn't!*

I'm going to share with you the **secret system** I've been teaching my patients since 1991.

Equally as important, it is the **same system** I use every day…

I LIVE WHAT I TEACH!

That wasn't always the case…

When I started 17 years ago at the

where I still currently work –

STRESS had *control* of me!

Only…

I didn't *realize* it...

It wasn't until I landed

in my doctor's office

3 weeks in a row

with **horrible migraines** & he asked

"Carol, what's got you so stressed?"

Now, the most **embarrassing** part:

Here I was *teaching my patients*

the

to manage their stress…

BUT I wasn't *using them myself!*

Since that day,

I have **kept** my commitment to

I LIVE WHAT I TEACH every day!

Everything I share here with you –

I use Myself!

About This Book

I doubt you have read a like this!

I like to use a lot of pictures, analogies, & word art which help information stick in the brain!

I call my approach:

SMARTheory™

(It's what makes my books and services *different* from all others!)

KNOWLEDGE is the *left brain* at work.

This is where YOU *know* what to do!

Since I use "pictures" & "images", I end up

tapping into the other side of the brain –

the right side!

With both sides working

on the same page,

the end result is getting people to

Move knowledge in to ACTION!

You'll find this book is broken in to 3 parts:

Part One: It's In The Cards!
Part Two: Now You See It!
Part Three: Now You Don't!

Part 1:

There will be **many** things having to do with your wedding that you'll want to **be your way!**

We'll look at **WHY** that may not always be possible.

Part 2:

Here I introduce you to a concept that will **CHANGE** your life **forever**….

 You'll never think about stress the same way **again!**

You also learn WHY *we must*

DO something about it.

Did you know…

Studies show over 80% of people

DO NOTHING about

their record high stress levels.

Part 3:

This section will **give** YOU the tools

to get the job done!

You'll learn **A LOT** of

different "tools"!

The secret I learned a long time ago…

Having the *right tool*

    for the *right job* makes

        the difference between

success and failure.

Also,

1 TOOL *won't work* the **same** for everyone!

Part One
It's In The Cards!

It's In The Cards!

When you come to my live seminars, as you take your seat, you'll be handed a playing card!

It may be a king or it may be a three....

The **key point** is:

You **DON'T** get to **CHOOSE** what card you get!

This applies so wonderfully **to LIFE** – where we'll face many situations that

WE DON'T GET TO CHOOSE!

When planning your wedding,

you may want to control everything….

However, **YOU CAN'T!**

Here are some tools I use with this:

> IT'S NOT
>
> *WHAT HAPPENS*
>
> TO YOU,
>
> BUT
>
> *HOW YOU REACT*
>
> TO IT
>
> **THAT MATTERS**
>
> EPICTETUS

Another way to think about it....

We don't get to control the events,

We *do get to control*

our response to them!

We are 100% responsible for our **choice:**

Controlling

How

Our

Intentions

Create

Experiences

© 2019 & licensed by Well YOUniversity, LLC
Taken from the *WordTools Series*

This is my favorite &

the *MOST* POWERFUL:

When we face a situation

that *CANNOT* be Changed

We are **CHALLENGED**

to

CHANGE OURSELVES

Victor Frankl

Are you trying to change things

you CAN'T CONTROL?

Do the exercise on the next page to see!

Write down as many things you can think of having to do with your wedding:

(Use another piece of paper if you need more room!)

Now go back & circle

ONLY the things **you can control!**

Tracking Your Progress

Monitoring

I developed a **tool** to help my patients be able to track their progress.

The Stressometer™

It's pretty simple to use!

1st - Read each question & select the answer that *best describes* you.

2nd - When you get to the end, *total up* all the numbers for a score

3rd - *Check your score* on the key. Repeat to see how you progress!

The Stressometer

I find when I try to go to sleep, my mind just keeps racing about things.

    1   2   3   4   5   6   7
Not at all   All the time

I find my appetite changes, I'm either eating more or eating less.

    1   2   3   4   5   6   7
Not at all   All the time

I find myself getting really angry over the littlest things.

    1   2   3   4   5   6   7
Not at all   All the time

I find I am having increased health issues. (ie. migraines, pain, & digestive)

    1   2   3   4   5   6   7
Not at all   All the time

I find my relationship is being impacted by what goes on at work / home.

    1   2   3   4   5   6   7
Not at all   All the time

Total: _____

How Stressed Are You?

5–10 **Great news!**
   You have no stress!

11–15 **Good news!**
   You have just a little bit of stress!

16–20 **Not bad!**
   You seem to still have a handle on it!

21–25 **WATCH OUT!**
   STRESS is *starting to cause trouble!*

26–30 **WARNING…**
   STRESS is *greatly impacting* your life.

31–35 **DANGER Zone!**
   Your level has you at extreme risk.

Your score *will come down* when you use the system!!!

Another Tracking Tool

How to tell if this is helping!

There are 2 more ways to track -

Both use a score of 1 to 100

#1 Track your **daily** stress level
(do this every evening)

#2 Track your level **before & after** you use the tools!

***Since this is new for you
it may take a little time for you to
get used to the tools!***

In order for this system to WORK…

YOU must *take* **ACTION!**

Here are a couple of my **WordTools** to help:

A

Critical

Task

Implemented

Only

Now!

© 2019 & licensed by Well YOUniversity, LLC
Taken from the *WordTools Series*

No "tool" will work…

      if you don't **pick it up**

              &

      DO something with it!!

Here's my WordTool:

Direct

Opportunity

© 2019 & licensed by Well YOUniversity, LLC
Taken from the *WordTools Series*

Lastly,

When we **_DON'T_** use the "tools"

This is what happens!

Denied

Opportunity

Not

'

Trying

© 2019 & licensed by Well YOUniversity, LLC
Taken from the *WordTools Series*

Part Two
Now You See It!
(Two ways to 'see' it!)

#1

Imagine this ...

I hand you a big bottle of root beer

and ask you to *shake it up –*

A LOT!

Maybe you even **drop**

it on the floor...

So,

what do you think will **happen**

to the bottle of root beer?

You're **right!**

The PRESSURE builds up inside!

And once *the pressure gets built up*

It stays there...

It won't go away on its own.

The PRESSURE doesn't go *anywhere*

we *do something to let it out!*

And, it's *not good* to have **too much** PRESSURE build up inside the bottle.

Two things can happen…

#1 It comes SPILLING OUT & leaves a big mess.

#2 It STAYS IN and ends up *ruining* the root beer.

It's best to avoid both!

People are like the bottle ...

Things happen in life that

shake a person up

And...

Just like the pressure
BUILT UP
in the bottle...

STRESS builds up *inside people!*

And once the *STRESS* gets built up

It stays there...

It won't go away on its own.

The **STRESS** doesn't go anywhere

we *do something to let it out!*

(we'll talk about this in part 2)

And just like the bottle,

It's *not good* for **too much**

STRESS to

build up inside people!

Here's what happens to people when **TOO MUCH** stress builds up…

#1   It comes SPILLING OUT & leaves a **big** mess.

Have you ever:

Said hurtful things or things you wished you hadn't said, yelled, got in a fight, broke things, or got in trouble at work or school?

#2   It STAYS IN and ends up ruining *your health.*

Have you ever:

Felt anxiety, can't sleep, gotten headaches, ate too much or not at all, felt sad & depressed, couldn't concentrate, worried a lot?

Do any of the following everyday life things **STRESS** you out?

Chronic Pain

    Bills / Finances

        Looking for work

           Being a caregiver

              Dr's appointments

              Holidays

Commute to work / school

    Relationships

        Not working

            Getting sick

              Family members

              Kids / Pets

Running late or waking up late

Important news:

A situation that *causes* one person stress

may not *cause* you stress!

Now, what are the wedding things

stressing you out?

Write them down here:

(Use another piece of paper if you need more room!)

#2

What do you think would happen if…

You **plugged** the drain,

> turned the water **on**,

>> and then *walked away*?

Eventually….

> It would **overflow**, right?

> Once it did – there'd be a

HUGE MESS!

Does this make sense?

A tub can only hold **so much!**

<u>Two important points:</u>

1) Once the level starts to rise – It will KEEP rising until it is **shut off.**

2) The tub ONLY has *so much room* - It can ONLY hold *so much* then it's

OVERFLOW!!!

Some people think…

The solution is to just **turn OFF the water.**

You'll see later why this *won't* work!

When it comes to ***STRESS…***

People are just like a tub:

1) Once you wake up –

your **STRESS** level starts to rise

& it will keep rising until it is…

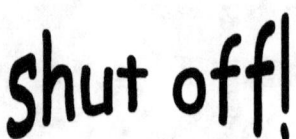

2) *YOU* only have *so much room* -

YOU can only hold so much

STRESS

until *YOU* will be at

OVERFLOW!!!

So,

I hope you can 👓 how

STRESS creates problems

And how it won't go away

until we…

release it!

Now that you can **SEE IT:**

Way #1

Way #2

It's time to learn how to

RELEASE IT!

We're moving on to Part Two…

Part Three
Now You Don't!
(Ways to 'release' it!)

What To Do!

This is where almost everyone

gets it **wrong!**

Because you're reading this book…

you'll know the

What you are about to learn is my *secret*

DO*60* System™

- ➢ It ***doesn't take*** a lot of ***time***!
- ➢ It will work for ***everyone***!
- ➢ It can be used ***everywhere***!

There are **2** steps to the

DO*60* System™

Step 1 -

the level from **RISING!**

Step 2 -

RELEASE so the level drops!

Each step must be done *in order...*

Step 1 ➡ Step 2

Each step must be done *for 60 Secs.*

Just so this makes sense...

In order to the level from **rising** you must do something that is

calming for you!

Calming = Activities that require

NO energy or muscles

be used!

I'm afraid I have a little bit of

 You can **ONLY** use your cell phone for this first step!

Cell phones *DO NOT* require

enough energy or muscles for Step Two.

Now,

In order to **release** & drop levels

you must do something *you like*

that is ACTIVE

Active = Activities that **DO** require

energy & muscles

BE USED!

So let's apply this to our stress bottle…

Step 1 - **the pressure**

from continuing to build up!

Step 2 - **the pressure**

that's been built up inside!

Each step:

- ✓ Must be done **in order**
- ✓ Must be done for **60 secs.**

** Otherwise the system won't work **

And applied to our stress tub…

Step 1 - **the level**

from continuing to rise!

Step 2 - **the level**

that's been raised already!

Where most people get it wrong…

They only *turn OFF the water.*

They **DON'T** do Step 2 - **RELEASE!**

How To Do It!
Step 1

Sign Up Today!

This 5 minute video newsletter will give you more tips, tools, & rules for taking control of…

STRESS!

Sign up at:

StressYOUniversity.com/Stress-Talk

On the following pages are

a bunch of different **"tools"**.

Each one is good to use for

Step 1 -

Things from **RISING!**

There are a **4 keys** to

S
  U
    C
      C
        E
          S
            S....

Try out each one.
(***even if*** you don't think it will work for you!)

 ## Do 60 Seconds.
(if you can go longer – ***do it!*** 30 secs. ***is better than*** none!)

 ## Keep a list.
(write down tools that end up working ***best for you***)

 ## Have more than 1!
(don't set yourself up to fail the ***more tools*** the better!)

You **must** do **Step 1** *before* Step 2

Step 1 ⟶ Step 2

Tool #1

read

grab one of your favorite books

Real   or   **Kindle**

Either way….. you're reading!

 Tool #2

Music

Listen to one of your favorites!

Song   or   **Artist**

Tool #3

Breathe

✓ **Count your breathes**

There are a couple ways to do this:

#1   **Track the # you do in 60 secs.**

or

#2   **Set a specific # to do 10, 12, 15, 20**

Belly Breathing is best!

This gets lots of oxygen in to our brain…

Oxygen is **kryptonite** to STRESS!

Another way to *BREATHE:*

✓ Square Breathing

1) **Breathe in** & count to 4 in your head (1,2,3,4)

2) **Hold it** & count to 4 in your head (1,2,3,4)

3) **Breathe out** & count to 4 in your head (1,2,3,4)

4) **Hold it** & count to 4 in your head (1,2,3,4)

5) **Repeat!**

Here's what it looks like!

Hold 1,2,3,4

In
1,2,3,4

Out
1,2,3,4

Hold 1,2,3,4

 **Tool #4**

Take A Time Out

Remove yourself from the situation.

Create between

YOU & the situation or person

Go outside!

**Go to
another room**

Tool #5

Mind Push Ups!

Here's how:

1. Find a quiet spot to lie down.

2. Set a timer for 60 secs. (*or more!*)

3. Put a book on your belly.

4. As you breathe in, make

   your belly & the book rise up!

5. Breathe out like your blowing candles.

6. Repeat breathes until timer goes off!

Tool #6

+ SELF-TALK

Saying positive statements to yourself!

The 2 P's of Self-Talk!

1) Present   FUTURE

   I AM…..   ~~I will….~~
   THIS IS….   ~~I hope…~~
   I HAVE….   ~~I'm going to…~~

2) Positive

   ~~Don't~~ touch = TOUCH!   ~~Not…~~
                              ~~Won't…~~
                              ~~Can't…~~

Our brain filters out the negative
& all we hear is what's after it: *TOUCH!*

** See a list of self-talk ideas on page 65 **

Tool #7

The Serenity Prayer

God,

Grant me the **serenity** to accept
                the things *I cannot change.*

The **courage** to change the things I *can.*

And the **wisdom** to know *the difference.*

Carol's
'In the Moment Serenity Prayer'

Ask yourself the following

"Can I do anything about IT

RIGHT NOW?"

If yes, ***DO it***!   If NO – ***Let it go!***

Here's a few more **tools –**

- Guided Imagery on

- Count to 10 **s l o w l y !**

- Watch a favorite show or movie

- Blow bubbles

- Lie down & look at the sky

- Picture a STOP sign in your mind

- Make a "Calm Jar" Google It!

Positive Self-Talk Ideas

I no longer give power to the PAST

Today I feel peace & calm.

I am free of negative feelings.

I am learning to love myself.

Today, I choose a positive attitude.

I am terrific just the way I am!

I have all the time I need.

I am living a healthy life today

Today, I forgive all others and myself.

I am getting there one step at a time!

I am having a great day!

I am a good friend to have!

Can you think of other ways for you to:

 The level from **RISING!**

(Use another piece of paper if you need more room!)

Remember -

This step is one that is calming...

(Requires NO activity or muscles!)

How To Do It!
Step 2

Now we'll take a look at what to do *once* you have done

Step 1

On the following pages are

more **"tools"**...

Each one of these is

good to use for

Step 2 -

RELEASE what's there!

Again, here are those 's to success!

#1 **Try out each one.**
    (*even if* you don't think
    It will work for you!)

#2 **Do 60 Seconds.**
    (if you can go longer – *do it!*
    30 secs. *is better than* none!

#3 **Keep a list.**
    (write down tools that end
    up working *best for you*)

#4 **Have more than 1!**
    (don't set yourself up to fail
    the *more tools* the better!)

Remember: you **must** do Step 1 *before* Step 2

    Step 1 ⟶ Step 2

Tool #1

Talk

Grab one of your favorite friends

In-person

Text

Phone

Either way….. You're *talking!*

IMPORTANT:

Talk about your *feelings*, **not** the situation!

Tool #2

Do A Dump & Destroy

This is one of my secret weapons!

Here's what you need:

- ✓ A piece of paper
- ✓ Something to write with

1) Start writing

2) *DO NOT* READ IT

3) *Destroy* IT!

It WON'T work with a computer
It requires you to use paper!

This is different from "Journaling"….

with Dumping –

The goal = Just **get it out!**
Reading IT = ***reloads*** *it!*

It also works *really well* when**…

1) You can't **fall asleep** because your *mind racing*

2) You **wake up** at night & your mind is racing!

**IMPORTANT:

You must go write in ***another*** room for it to work.

TIP: Use a sharpie & toilet paper, flush when done. No one will ever read that!

Tool #3
Empty Chair Method

When you don't have anyone

or you can't get a hold of someone

 this tool!

You start talking to the

"Empty Chair"

As if the person was there!

It is a great way to VENT without

getting in trouble for what you say!

Tool #4

Get ACTIVE!

There are many ways to do this!

Walk

Any Kind of Exercise

 Climb the Stairs

 Bike

Push Ups

Sports

Tool #5

Music

For this tool to work, you MUST:

you **DO more** than just listen!

Dance = Any time you are moving to music!

sing = Doesn't mean you *can* or **KNOW** the words!

Perform = Play a real instrument

or

AIR guitar / drums

Tool #6

Punch n Dump!

There are **2** ways to do this:

1) Use a real punching bag.

Don't have one?

You can make one using a pillow!

 +

2) Air Boxing!

You must ***be sure*** to do this in a

place where it is SAFE.

Tool #7

Let It Out!

When stress builds up…

Sometimes a good cry or a good laugh is needed to ***let it out!***

 It's perfectly okay to let the tears flow.

 (Even for guys)

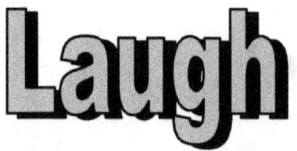 Watch a funny show

Try Laughter Yoga

Here's a few more ***tools –***

- Tear up an old phone book or a bunch of paper

- Wash the car

- Do some coloring!

- Clean the house!

- Do some jumping jacks!

- Scream in a car or another safe place

- Constructive Destruction – break something on PURPOSE!

Can you think of other ways for you to:

 RELEASE what's there!

(Use another piece of paper if you need more room!)

Remember -

This step is one that is *active*...

(DOES require activity or muscles!)

Wrap Up!

Congratulations!

You now have the "tools" to become a

Stress Master!

More importantly,

    You can now MANAGE

        your **wedding stress!**

So here's what we've covered:

Part 1: It's In The Cards!

You don't always get to be in

control of things...

Sometimes,

 You just must play the cards you get.

YOU are **100% responsible**

for *your response!*

Part 2: Now You See It!

So,

There are **2** ways I got you to

 STRESS

Way # 1

Things happen in life that
shake a person up

And…

Just like the pressure
BUILT UP
in the bottle…

STRESS builds up *inside people!*

And once the *STRESS gets built up*

It stays there...

It won't go away on its own.

The **STRESS** doesn't go anywhere

we *do something to*

Let

   It

      Out!

Way #2

People are just like a tub:

1) Your **STRESS** level starts to rise & it will keep rising until it is…

shut off!

2) *YOU* only have *so much room* - *YOU* can only hold so much

STRESS

until *YOU* will be at

OVERFLOW!!!

And how it won't go away

until we…

release it!

Part 2: Now You Don't!

There are **2** steps to the

DO*60* System™

Step 1 -

the level from **RISING!**

Step 2 -

RELEASE so the level drops!

➢ **Each step** must be done *in order...*

Step 1 ➡ Step 2

➢ **Each step** must be done *60 Secs.*

Remember:

Most everyone in the world

gets it **wrong!**

They don't know to **DO** Step 2

Now you know the secret!

Bonus Tool

I created this tool for my patients & **discovered** I **needed** it more!

If you start ***feeling overwhelmed,***

I want you to use this:

The Serenity Prayer Stress Tool!

#1 Make a list of ALL the things that are stressing you out.

#2 Using the worksheet on the next page, place the things from your list in the appropriate section.

#1 Fold the paper on the line and RIP IT IN HALF. Get rid of what you CAN'T do anything about!

I have also created a couple

mini posters!

This way you can rip / cut them out of the book

And put them up on your fridge, computer, or wherever you'll see them!

This will help reinforce the new tools you're trying to get good at using!

The Serenity Pryer Stress Tool!

Grant me the **serenity** to accept the things I cannot change:

_____

_____

_____

_____

- - - - - - - - - - - - - - - - - -

The **courage** to change the things I can:

_____

_____

_____

_____

And the **wisdom** to know the difference!

Intentionally blank

DO*60* System™-

Step 1 -   *NO* Muscles

the level from **RISING!**

Step 2 -   *NEEDS* Muscles

RELEASE so the level drops!

> **Each step** must be done *in order...*

Step 1 ➡ Step 2

> **Each step** must be done *60 Secs...*

Intentionally blank

The 's to success!

 #1 Try out each one.
(***even if*** you don't think it will work for you!)

 #2 Do 60 Seconds.
(if you can go longer – ***do it!*** 30 secs. ***is better than*** none!)

#3 Keep a list.
(write down tools that end up working ***best for you***)

 #4 Have more than 1!
(don't set yourself up to fail the ***more tools*** the better!)

The Stressometer

I find when I try to go to sleep, my mind just keeps racing about things.

　1　　2　　3　　4　　5　　6　　7
Not at all   All the time

I find my appetite changes, I'm either eating more or eating less.

　1　　2　　3　　4　　5　　6　　7
Not at all   All the time

I find myself getting really angry over the littlest things.

　1　　2　　3　　4　　5　　6　　7
Not at all   All the time

I find I am having increased health issues. (ie. migraines, pain, & digestive)

　1　　2　　3　　4　　5　　6　　7
Not at all   All the time

I find my relationship is being impacted by what goes on at work / home.

　1　　2　　3　　4　　5　　6　　7
Not at all   All the time

Total: _____

**Use key – page 14

Want to Speed Up Your Progress?

Join Carol for this

FREE Special Training

for brides!

™

You know the **DO60** System –

Now it's time to learn the 5 keys to

being an unstoppable Stress Master!

Sign Up Now!

StressYOUniversity.com/Mastery

Sign Up For

This 5 minute video newsletter will give you more tips, tools, & rules for taking control of...

STRESS!

Sign up at:

StressYOUniversity.com/Stress-Talk

Carol's Other Resources

A Nationally Syndicated Wellness Series:

The WELL YOU Show

Mondays @ 6pm, Sundays @ 8am

Watch at: www.PrincetonTV.org

Catch past episodes at
www.TheWellYouShow.com

Want More Tools?!

Carol has written more "tool" books!

If you need help:

- ✓ Losing weight
- ✓ Dealing with anger
- ✓ Managing health issues

Take a look at the next few pages…

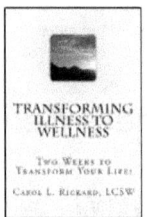 Chronic illness doesn't exclude you from having wellness. Get a blueprint to follow for taking back control of your health!

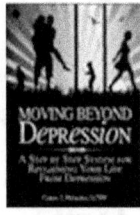 Are you sick & tired of feeling sick & tired? This is a step by step system for reclaiming your life from depression.

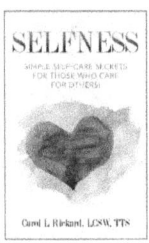 Self-care is often forgotten in this busy world. Carol offers simple and practical strategies to fit in to your busy life!

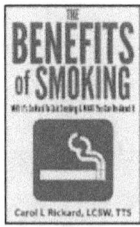 No – this is not promoting smoking! Instead, it provides the knowledge & the 'tools' to finally "Kick Cigarettes Butts"!

Available: amazon.com/author/carolrickard

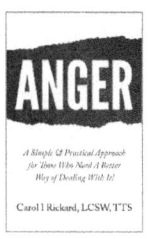

ANGER - one of the most powerful emotions there is. Learn how to manage it instead of it managing you!

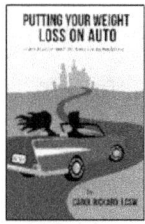

Losing weight doesn't have to be complicated! Learn the 7 Laws of Lasting Weight Loss a car can teach us. Guaranteed to work!

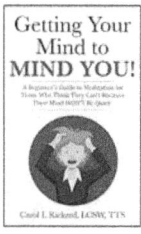

Your mind *is not* supposed to be quiet! Learn how mediation really works & change your life forever!

Do you find yourself struggling with what to say or how to help someone you care about? Learn how to say it & what to do!

Available: amazon.com/author/carolrickard

WordTools

What are words tools?
They are acronyms with purpose & meaning!

They are officially called *Artinyms™*, which is Sanskrit for "describe".

On the back of each wordtool is a question for you to answer should you choose to!

We have **4 different versions:**

Wellness Vol. 1 & 2,   *Self-Esteem* Vol. 1 & 2
Business Vol. 1 & 2,   *Athletes* Vol. 1

Examples:

The
Only
Day
Afforded
You!

A
Deliberate
Adjustment
Providing
Transformation

Daringly
Recognize
Experiences
As
Mine

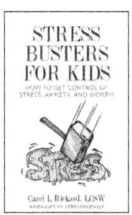

NEW RELEASE!!!!
Kid these days have to deal with so much stress. This makes sure they have the tools to succeed!!

We have three different versions of adult stress books because life circumstances can be different for each..

Choose the one that *best fits* your situation!

Caregiver

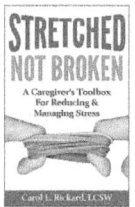

Research has shown caregivers are the MOST vulnerable. Learn quick, simple, practical tools for reducing and managing it.

Stress Eater

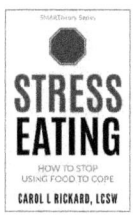

Do you find yourself eating when under stress? Get the tools & knowledge needed to break away from any old habits.

General

STRESS... It's all around us and NOT getting any less! Get the system Carol has taught to 1,000's & finally take control!

To Contact Carol:

Please feel free to reach out if you have questions or comments!

Email:

Carol@StressYOUniversity.com

Phone:

888 LifeTools

(543-3866)

Sign Up for Stress Talk:

StressYOUniversity.com/Stress-Talk

www.ingramcontent.com/pod-product-compliance
Lightning Source LLC
LaVergne TN
LVHW020936090426
835512LV00020B/3379